EFT

EFT TAPPING SCRIPTS & SOLUTIONS TO AN ABUNDANT YOU

10 Simple DIY Experiences To Prove That Your Mind Creates Your Life!

JANET EVANS

EFT: EFT Tapping Scripts & Solutions To An Abundant YOU

10 Simple DIY Experiences To Prove That Your Mind Creates Your Life!

Janet Evans

Contents

Introduction 3

Chapter 1 – Discovering the Emotional Freedom Technique 4

Chapter 2 – EFT tapping scripts: What are they and how are they performed? 12

Chapter 3 – 10 simple DIY experiences to prove that your mind creates your life 18

Conclusion 30

Introduction

A new psychological treatment method known as the Emotional Freedom Technique (EFT) has been gaining in popularity all over the world nowadays. After all, many people who have tried this technique attest to the fact that it is effective in helping solve some of the common problems that people are experiencing.

In this book, this technique will be discussed further. Its unique features – tapping our meridian points and using scripts to deal with the problem – will be presented along with sample scripts to get you started with the practice.

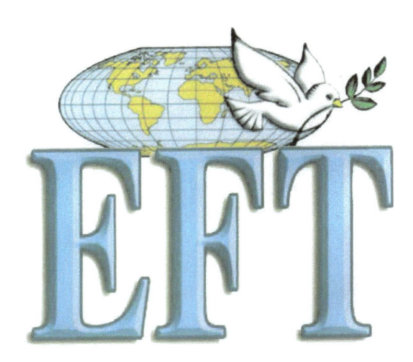

Chapter 1 – Discovering the Emotional Freedom Technique

A new method that is drawing attention today when it comes to helping individuals cope with their problems is EFT or the Emotional Freedom Technique. In this chapter, we will discuss the basics of this revolutionary therapy method.

What is EFT?

Emotional Freedom Techniques (EFT) was a method created by Gary Craig in his EFT Handbook published in the late 1990s. It is a relatively new treatment method under Energy Psychology, combining many different methods such as acupuncture (a Chinese traditional treatment approach), neuro-linguistic programming, Thought Field Therapy, and energy medicine.

Also referred to as "psychological acupressure," this technique is aimed at helping individuals to live their lives harmoniously by unblocking the energy system – this is believed to be the source of emotional discomforts. These blockages are also believed to limit our beliefs and behaviors. This manifests in the form of different emotional and physical problems such as depression and anxiety, lack of self-esteem and confidence, and a higher risk of adopting addictive and compulsive behaviors. After all, it is now believed that some physical symptoms can be causes of emotional disharmonies. This led to the technique being an acceptable form of treatment, and it is now being used in the fields of psychotherapy and medicine.

How does it work?

Generally, EFT works through the use of "tapping" energy meridian points while mentioning affirmative phrases. As this technique was influenced by acupuncture, these energy meridian points throughout the body are already determined; the only difference is that EFT doesn't need to use needles in order to accomplish the desired effect. EFT only uses the fingertips to input kinetic energy in these meridians (primarily on the head and chest) while you're thinking of a specific problem that you want to have solved and voicing out positive affirmations while "tapping." In short, you are unblocking the meridian points of negative energy and the verbalizing of positive affirmations serve as the replacement of those you have removed. By doing so, you are stuffing your meridian points (and ultimately your whole system) with positive energy. This restores physical and psychological balance, and makes healing faster.

When should it be done?

For you to get the full effects of tapping in your life, you should do it as often as you can. Generally, the practice should be done upon waking up, before you take your meals, when you need to go to the bathroom, and before you go to bed.

It is also advised that if possible, you should apply it even in public situations such as when you are waiting for the traffic light to turn green, or when you're seated on your office chair. However, doing it in public has one major flaw – it is too conspicuous and looks awkward. In these cases, you can only use at least two fingers on one hand for tapping. With this practice, you can continue with your tapping without looking awkward or having other people's attention directed to you.

Tapping techniques

The following are important tapping techniques that you should use in order to ensure that you are doing it properly and will therefore gain the full benefits from it:

1. In order to maximize the benefits that you can get from tapping, it is important that you use all your fingertips in tapping the meridian points. During the early development of the technique, only two fingers were initially used for tapping. As it went through changes, the use of four fingertips is now being implemented and taught to patients. This is for the reason that the use of four fingertips will cover a larger area than tapping with just one or two fingers. Also, it will be easier for you to cover the meridian points (although it is not necessary to hit the meridian points precisely unlike in acupuncture).

2. Use your fingertips, not your finger pads. This is for the reason that your fingertips have more meridian points than the finger pads. Finger pads may only be used by women who have long fingernails.

3. Remove any accessories such as watches, bracelets, or glasses as they can interfere with the technique. Although you can go around the accessories while tapping, you will be able to cover a good portion of the meridian points if your accessories are removed.

4. Apply enough pressure while tapping – just enough to make the pressure felt by your body or face, but not hard enough that it will hurt you while tapping.

How to find the right tapping points

Aside from the significance of the fingertips in the whole EFT process, you should also know the specific areas where you should tap. The meridian points in this list are presented in order (This is the sequence that you should follow while doing the technique.).

1. Start with the top of your head. Specifically, you should tap from the center of the skull going down to the upper part of the back of your head.

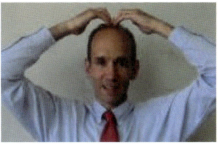

2. From the top of the head, do the tapping on the beginning of your eyebrows, following the part just above the area covered by your eyebrows. Spread your fingers thoroughly, with your pinky fingers almost meeting each other on the center of your face (on top of your nose).

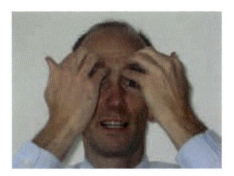

3. From your eyebrows, you should tap on the side of the eyes. This refers to the bone where your eyes are located.

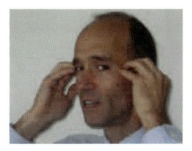

4. Move the tapping under the eyes. This is the part under the bone where the eyes are located. Specifically, this is the area just above the cheeks and is near the nostrils.

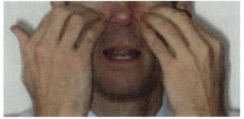

5. From under the eyes, tap on the area under the nose. Specifically, this refers to the area where you grow your moustache (just below the nostrils and near the top of your upper lip.

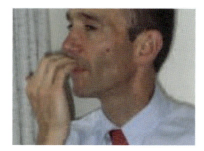

6. After the tapping under the nose, you should next tap your chin (or your chin point). This refers to the area below your bottom lip, in the middle of your chin area.

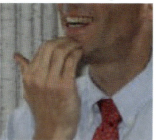

7. From the chin area, the tapping should be moved onto the collar bone area. In order to locate this area (as the collar bone in this context is different from the real collar bone in our anatomy), first locate the U-shaped portion found on the bottom of the neck (where you get to touch the bone in the middle of the chest). From the U-shaped bone, move down an inch lower it and move an inch to either side (left or right). This is referred to as the collar bone.

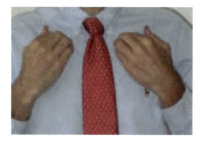

8. From the collar bone, move on to the area under the arm. This is found on the side of the body, at around 4 inches below your armpit. For men, this is the area found on the side of the nipples; for women, this area is found on the middle of their bra straps.

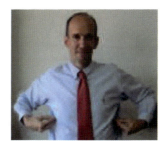

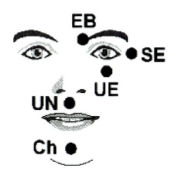

TH = Top of Head
EB = Eye Brow
SE = Side of the Eye
UE = Under the Eye
UN = Under the Nose
Ch = Chin
CB = Collar Bone
UA = Under the Arm

This figure aims to point out the areas in our body that should be tapped and their sequence. Along with it would be the specific areas in the face that should be tapped.

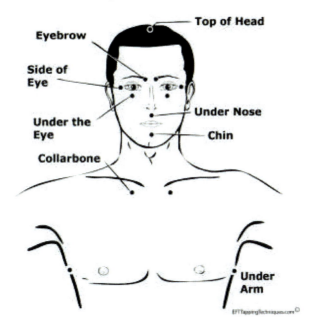

This figure shows in detail the 8 tapping points for the whole body.

What benefits can tapping give you?

Tapping is found out to produce benefits on the following conditions:

- It was found out to improve your health and/or influence your health habits such as the following:

- a. Helps in relieving pain
- b. It can help you to relax and accommodate sleep (hence overcoming insomnia).
- c. Can influence your emotions and its link to your diet; this includes helping you to reduce or eliminate food or substance cravings, or can help to eliminate emotions that may be preventing you from adapting a healthy lifestyle.

- It can serve as a supplementary treatment for the following psychological diseases or emotions:
  - a. Can help reduce the occurrence of stress and anxiety
  - b. Can help reduce frustrations, depression, and anger
  - c. Can help you to get rid of guilt feelings and get over traumatic experiences
  - d. Can serve as a relaxation technique in conjunction with treatment for all kinds of phobias and fears
  - e. It can also be used along with psychotherapy methods for addiction, and mood and personality disorders
  - f. Can help to address different issues such as those related to yourself (confidence or self-esteem) and of your relationships

- It could increase your performance or effectiveness in the following situations:
  - a. Sports
  - b. Improve confidence and other skills that can be used for the advancement of your career; this includes the improvement of your communication skills (especially if you have problems with public speaking or with presenting to a large number of people), improving your professional relationships, and having an open mind on the expansion of your career (taking risks with your money in order to start your own business)

- Improve the overall quality of life through the following:
  - a. Learn how to muster up your courage and try to do the things that you wanted to accomplish a long time ago yet you never did because of your apprehension
  - b. Learning to release any emotions that can hinder you from experiencing a more enjoyable life

The Pros and Cons of tapping

Tapping, as a part of EFT, generally brings benefits to practitioners. However, it also has some problems.

Pros

1. Tapping is safe and pain-free; this is because tapping does not use needles as compared to acupuncture. Also, it does not require the use of any drugs unlike to other forms of therapy (where drugs can be used in conjunction with other psychotherapies). Therefore, no side effects will be experienced.

2. Tapping is also cost-efficient; anyone who can comprehend from the free videos or written instructions on how it can be done correctly will be able to apply it on themselves with minimal supervision.

3. It can be considered as effective, since many people who have tried this technique have testified that it produces positive results.

Cons

1. One major drawback of this method is that even if there are a significant number of people who attest to its effectiveness, it's still not considered as an actual therapy method in the same league as drugs or older forms of psychotherapy. Hence, it can be concluded that the method may not be reliable enough for it to be considered as an actual treatment for its target disorders.

2. Since many people can apply it to themselves because it is a cost-efficient method, they may not consult with "real" professionals anymore. They may just result to "self-medication" instead of seeking a more reliable form of therapy for their disorder/illness.

3. Since tapping is not considered as an actual therapy method, it cannot be regulated by the government. Hence, there are no real accredited professionals who practice it. There may be groups that can give certifications to people and refer to them as "experts," but always keep in mind that certification is more lenient than regulation. Hence, the government will not be able to protect the interest of "clients" from those who claim that they are experts in the field.

4. The practice of tapping may take a longer time before any effects can be seen, even with the fact that the individuals doing the treatment themselves are aware of their condition, are motivated to change, and are cooperative with the system. Some people might even think that the technique only gives false hope to those who are adapting it as a treatment method.

Tapping is only one half of the whole system of the Emotional Freedom Technique. Since it is a painless way to unblock your meridian points of negative energy, it is preferred over acupuncture by a significant number of people (even if the latter delivers benefits at a much faster rate and is considered as an alternative and effective form of treatment). With tapping already discussed, we can now go to the second half of EFT.

Chapter 2 – EFT tapping scripts: What are they and how are they performed?

Tapping, as the first half of the Emotional Freedom Techniques, was discussed in the previous chapter. However, in order to make this behavior produce significant effects on the individual, the second half – or the tapping scripts – should also be applied. In this chapter, we will talk about this method as well as the process on how it is performed.

What are tapping scripts?

A tapping script is an affirmative line that usually accompanies your tapping behavior. As mentioned in the previous chapter, it is the tapping that unblocks our meridian points of negative energy. This is the role of the tapping script. To replace the negative energy you once had with a positive one, something positive should be present while the tapping is taking place. In this case, that "something positive" is the affirmative phrase.

How is it applied?

In conjunction with tapping, this is how EFT is applied:

1. First determine the negative emotions, issues, or problems that you want to address. It would be best if you can specify more than one problem, or if you can break down the general problem into specific issues.

2. After determining the problem, you need to rate each problem depending on its severity (with 10 being extreme or most severe and 0 being non-existent).

3. Specify your setup phrase – the setup phrase is the statement of the problem that you want to solve, and an affirmation that you still accept yourself even if you have such weakness. A common setup phrase would be "Even though (state your problem), I completely and totally love, accept, and forgive myself."

4. Repeatedly mention your setup phrase while tapping your karate chop point. This is the soft area found on the side of either hand, and is located just below your little finger. You may tap around seven times for each side (although counting is not really necessary).

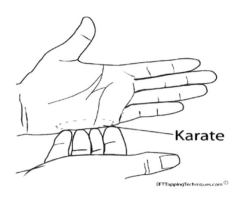

This figure shows the Karate chop point of the hands

5. Specify a reminder phrase – as the name suggests, this phrase serves as the reminder of the setup phrase that you pointed out during the earlier step. The reminder phrase is the one that should be spoken aloud while you go through with tapping the meridian points one after another.

6. After you've finished with the last meridian point, evaluate the problem once again. Gauge the level of discomfort that you have after one round of tapping, applying the 0-10 scale you used earlier.

7. Tapping should be repeated until such time that the rating for the problem is at least 2 or lower.

8. On the last round of tapping, you can change your setup phrases into more positive ones, especially now that the once-severe problem is not that severe anymore. You may add statements such as "I'm free of this problem" or "This problem doesn't bother me as much as it did before."

How can you make your own tapping script?

An individual's situation is as unique as the individual himself. Even when your negative emotions seem similar to others, yours will always be different. You may ask other people about their tapping scripts (if you have the same problem) or search the internet for scripts, but the therapy and meditation will only work best if what you're reciting is reflective of your situation.

The guidelines listed below may be followed if you want to make your own tapping script for each issue that you want to address.

1. After you specify the negative emotion that you want to work on, try to describe in detail the situation that led to the experience of that emotion.

2. From the previous step, give a detailed description of how the situation affected you on that same moment.

3. Similarly, describe in detail how that experience affected you now.

4. After step 3, you will have to give a detailed description of the negative outcomes that you have experienced during the time that the situation happened. Along with it, you also need to point out the negative outcomes that it is giving you up to this day.

5. Give a detailed description of what you feel about the outcomes brought by the situation.

6. Along with the past and present and negative outcomes, try to imagine the possible negative outcomes that you might experience in the future because of that situation. From these future outcomes, also give a detailed description of your feelings towards it.

7. Lastly, describe in detail what it is that you will do in order to change the situation if you have the chance or the ability to do so.

By following the steps stated above, you will be able to produce your own tapping script. Also, it will help you to determine what it is that really causes the emotional distress. This in turn will help you to devise methods that you may employ in order to solve the problem. After all, a problem can only be solved fully if you are aware of everything about it – from its source to the circumstances that maintain it.

Tips on how you can improve your affirmations

Affirmation is one of the key elements that made EFT an effective form of therapy. And if you want to maximize the benefit that you can get from affirmations, you should learn to apply certain practices in order to improve them. You may achieve this goal by adapting the following tips:

1. Learn how to properly time your affirmations – in order for you to experience the effects of EFT at a much faster rate, it is important that you develop the habit of tapping and affirmation, specifically at certain times of the day. In this manner, you won't miss a day without doing EFT. It is said that the best times to deliver your affirmations are during the following:

    a. When you wake up – since you are preparing for the day ahead, you have to tell yourself something positive in order for your system to respond in the same manner.

b. Every time you go to the bathroom – going for a bathroom break is similar to taking a break from your current situation. This is also the time when you can go and refresh or touch yourself up. With this in mind, tapping and affirmation are useful in the sense that they help you to continue with the task that you have to accomplish for that day with renewed positivity in mind. When you get back from the bathroom, you will continue to be at your best in whatever it is that you're doing.

c. Before going to sleep – tired as you may be, you should still take the time to tap and affirm yourself before you rest in your bed. With affirmation, it helps you to end your day on a positive note. Also, the positive thought will be processed by your brain during sleep, making your subconscious mind work on the affirmations while you're resting. When you wake up, your body will have adapted to the positive thought that you've had the previous night and ultimately influence the body to apply it during the day.

2. Deliver your affirmations while looking in the mirror – if you have some time on your hands for EFT, delivering your affirmations will be more effective if you do it while looking at yourself in the mirror. This is because the delivery will be much more direct if you're looking at your own reflection while listening to it rather than just listening to it alone. It's as if you are outside yourself, and saying the affirmation directly to yourself. This technique becomes easier to apply if you develop the habit of delivering affirmations and tapping when you go to the bathroom (since most bathrooms have mirrors).

3. Consistently affirm yourself and be patient with the results – affirmations can be awkward (or even funny) to hear at first. After all, it is something that was never a part of your system before. However, for the affirmation to happen and be adopted by your body, you have to deliver it on a regular basis. It may not produce any noticeable result at first, but it should not be taken as a sign that you should stop with affirming yourself. Rather, it should be thought of as an opportunity for you to continue with the affirmation. In time, there will be a noticeable change with regard to your goal or the problem that you want to solve. Continue with your affirmations – you will never know when this seed will grow and bear fruit.

4. Turn your fears into positive affirmations – it is inevitable that your fears will be touched while doing the technique; after all, the tapping scripts require you to specify the issues that you want to deal with. Hence, you should turn those fears into positive affirmations – and this is possible only if you acknowledge their existence. Writing it down on a piece of paper will help remind you that you should work on it while tapping, and it will help you to devise an appropriate tapping script for it. By

acknowledging the fear instead of denying or avoiding it, your mind and body will be able to adjust accordingly to it and hopefully find the best solution in overcoming the fear.

5. Deliver your affirmations in the present tense – this is because if the affirmation is delivered in the future tense (statements such as "I will..."), your mind will consider it as something that you can accomplish at a much later time. On the other hand, if the affirmation is addressed in the present tense, your mind will be conditioned that change should be started immediately or NOW.

What makes the whole EFT process successful?

The whole EFT process involves the presence of both tapping the energy meridian points and the delivery of affirmation phrases. Here are the specific elements that really make it possible for the method to be successful:

1. EFT fosters love for yourself – one element that is also present in EFT (as with all other therapy methods) is that it helps you to learn how to accept yourself regardless of your strengths and weaknesses. EFT emphasizes that by accepting who you are, it will be easier for you to work on the solutions for these issues. This is because if you continue to criticize yourself for your shortcomings, you are restricting yourself and limiting the areas that you should have been exploring.

2. EFT is about give and take – in order for your mind and body to produce positivity, the same should also be given to it. This explains why this technique includes affirmation in its whole process; if you continuously deliver positive affirmation, your body and mind will give back the same response in return and give positive results in your life.

3. EFT tries to initiate forgiveness – along with self-acceptance, EFT also includes in its script that you still forgive yourself even if you have these weaknesses. This is because if you learn how to forgive, you also learn how to let go of the past. After all, it is difficult to start fresh and move forward if there's something that is binding you to a heavy burden and is preventing you from going on.

4. EFT helps you to develop your language – after all, words are considered as an expression and the extension of your thoughts. EFT helps you in learning how to deliver positive language since you won't be able to produce positive thoughts, actions, and changes if your language is not the same as your desired result. Also, it helps you to adapt other changes in the way you deliver your sentences such as learning how to own your words ("I choose...") or delivering in the present tense ("I am now...").

Along with the tapping technique presented before, the addition of scripts and affirmative statements makes the whole process of EFT more effective in implementing changes to people's thoughts and behavior. Just like any habit, it would be best if you can practice these methods (both tapping and affirmative statements) as often as you can in your daily life to experience its benefits much sooner.

Chapter 3 – 10 simple DIY experiences to prove that your mind creates your life

To help you get started with the practice of EFT, this chapter will provide you with sample tapping scripts that you can use in order to address some issues or emotions that you might have. Feel free to change them depending on your situation.

Relieving anxiety and stress

Anxiety and stress will always be felt by individuals as long as they're alive – and this is normal. However, too much of these two can produce a variety of problems that can limit your overall performance.

Before you start with the session, you have to first determine the cause of your anxiety and/or stress (as both can be caused by different reasons). This will be the starting point of your setup phrase (See sample provided in the previous chapter.).

Here is an example of one round of tapping along with the corresponding script:

- Setup phrase: Even if I am not excited about going to work (or school) because it gets me stressed out and the people there know how to make my day hard, I completely love and accept myself (Say this while tapping your karate chop point for 7 to 10 times. Afterwards, start reciting your reminder phrases while tapping in order the meridian points stated in the previous chapter.).

- Top of the Head (TH) – I am anxious about going to work/school.

- Eyebrow (EB) - I feel nervous.

- Side of the eye (SE) – Those people sure know how to ruin my day.

- Under the eye (UE) – The stress that this situation's causing me is too much for me to handle.

- Under the nose (UN) – I am surrounded with so much negative energy.

- Chin (Ch) – These people are pulling me down.

- Collarbone (CB) – And they are the cause of my anger and frustration.

- Under the arm (UA) – I think I am not in total control of the situation.

- Top of the Head – After all, I am experiencing all of this because of them.

This ends the first round of tapping. Now, take a deep breath and try to let go of the anxiety from your mind and body. Evaluate the intensity level of the emotional level using the 0 to 10 scale introduced in the previous chapter. Repeat by doing another round of tapping and evaluating your anxiety. If it goes lower than two, you can now start to reframe your reminder phrases and change the previously negative phrases into positive ones:

- TH – What if there's a way to let go of this anxiety?
- EB – Wouldn't it be nice if I can get rid of this nervousness?
- SE – Starting from this moment, everything they say or do will not hurt me anymore.
- UE – They don't hold the power to dictate what I should feel.
- UN – I now know how to release this stress.
- Ch – And I'm aiming to find peace.
- CB – I want to find balance and calmness.
- UA – I am not adopting their negativity as I want to see the best in any situation.
- TH – I deserve to feel calm and relaxed; hence, I am letting go of this anxiety.

You are free to add positive affirmations even if you've reached the last meridian point. You just need to start over from the top of the head. After all, there's no need to rate this round anymore.

Overcoming resistance to change

Even if it's true that change is the only constant thing in this world, some people are not comfortable when this happens. After all, change can go either way – it can be a change for the better or a change for the worse. Hence, some people prefer to have things unchanged. This provides them comfort and security. However, being resistant to change is also bad in that you will never take any opportunity that will improve your overall life. In these situations, you can apply this sample tapping script if you're the type of person who wants to overcome this resistance.

Here is a sample script that you can use in order to get started with EFT for this issue.

- Setup phrase: Even if I'm the type of person who refuses to adapt to change, I completely love and accept myself (tapping on the karate chop point).
- TH – I refuse to feel better and improve myself.

- EB – I refuse to forgive and let this go.
- SE – Whom will I blame if I did?.
- UE – I might be in pain and in suffering.
- Ch – But the familiarity gives me security.
- CB – You can never make me change.
- UA – After all, changing is hard and dangerous.
- TH – You may want to change me, but I don't want to change myself.

One unique feature of this script is that it tries to invoke change in an individual by making them see that staying as you are and being fearful of change will never result in the improvement of your current situation. And since most people wouldn't want to imagine getting stuck in this seemingly endless loop, they will immediately make a way to avoid it. This is especially useful if you somehow want to force yourself into solving or changing a problem or negative emotion that has been present for quite some time.

Tapping through your past

As mentioned in the previous chapter, one element that makes EFT successful is because it helps individuals learn how to let go of the past and move on with their lives. This script can help you in getting rid of the burden that may be preventing you from moving forward.

- Setup phrase: (while tapping the karate chop point) Even if it is painful to recall my past failures, it is worse to know that these same experiences are preventing me from getting close to the success that I want to achieve, now and in the future. It would be better if I have the power to start all over again.
- TH – I have failed in the past.
- EB – I was the loser in almost everything that I did.
- SE – These failures were the proof of such.
- UE – I always experience a long losing streak.
- UN – Regardless of the effort that I give to my work…
- Ch – all of these will always end in failure.
- CB – These failures always remind me…

- UA – ...to never push myself too hard...
- TH – because in the end, all these efforts will be in vain.

Relax for a while after you have finished one round of tapping. Afterwards, evaluate your feelings towards the issue. Resume with more rounds of tapping if your rating is not lower than two. After the succeeding rounds and upon reaching a rating of 2 or lower, recite your positive affirmations.

- TH – I am keeping my mind open about these failures...
- EB – ...and I am thankful that I've experienced them.
- SE – I am using them as stepping stones for success...
- UE – ...as they taught me what are the things that I should avoid...
- UN – ...and I choose to believe that failures in what I do ...
- Ch – ...don't mean that I myself am a failure.
- CB – I know that I'm capable of reaching greater heights...
- UA – ...by turning my past failures into lessons that will guide me to success.
- TH – I am welcoming success with open arms.

Feel free to add specific events where you've experienced failure in this script.

Healing your body and relieving physical pain

Nobody wants to experience pain. If you're currently experiencing it, you would want the sensation to go away as soon as possible. The tapping script for this issue focuses on helping you determine where the pain in your body is emanating; by doing so, you will get to focus your energy more in containing the pain, increase your threshold for it, and give you an idea about what may be causing the pain.

You may use this tapping script as a sample. Feel free to customize this sample based on what you're feeling:

- Setup phrase: Even if I'm experiencing this pain, I am accepting it with all my heart.
- TH – This pain that I'm feeling...
- EB – ...is there whether I like it or not...

- SE – I have to pay attention...
- UE – ...if it's changing or moving...
- UN – ...so that I will know...
- Ch – ...where I should focus my energy...
- CB – ...and what is the real reason...
- UA – ...behind this pain...
- TH – ...that I know only I can bear.

The pain may not subside because of tapping, but delivering affirmations will condition your mind and getting it ready can make the pain easier to bear.

Solving your craving through the help of tapping

This particular issue may be one of the most difficult to solve. This is because food is something that is hard to resist – after all, the body has the need for the nourishment that food provides. Hence, you have to make a conscious effort to determine if what you're feeling is legitimate hunger (if your body really needs to eat) or if the hunger is just because of your cravings. The scripts can also remind you of foods that you like, making it harder for you to cease thinking of it and may hinder your focus. And lastly, you have to be mindful of the venue where you will practice this technique. After all, it would be very hard for you to implement what you want to happen when you did the tapping inside the washroom of your favorite restaurant.

Upon following the conditions stated above, you can now follow these steps and apply this sample tapping script.

- Tapping should be done when you are currently experiencing the craving or if you know that you will be experiencing the craving anytime soon (if you typically experience the craving in a specific situation such as when work is too stressful). You should also evaluate the severity of the craving prior to tapping so that you can have baseline data of the experience (This will mostly be high; however, specify the severity of your craving for it.). Upon determining the rating, you can start with your tapping.

- Setup phrase: Even if I'm currently experiencing this ___ craving (severity of the craving) for ___ (Specify the name of the food that you're craving for.), I completely love and accept myself anyway.

- TH – This craving...

- EB – …is keeping me preoccupied…
- SE – …even if I know…
- UE – …that I can survive without it…
- UN – …and it made me hate my body…
- Ch – …because I have ____ (if there is any health condition such as high blood pressure or sugar) due to too much consumption.
- CB – I lost the confidence to deal with other people…
- UA – …and it held me back…
- TH – …because I can't do the things that I used to accomplish before.

Evaluate if your craving has subsided. If it did, you can change your setup phrase to "Even if I still have this ____ craving for ____, I completely love and accept myself anyway." This acknowledgement serves as reinforcement to continue with another round of tapping and reciting the scripts until the craving is significantly diminished. For the final round, your affirmations while tapping should focus on the actions that you will be taking in order to suppress the craving.

Tapping script for creating love and a healthy relationship

Developing a tapping script for a relationship is not an easy task; this is because a healthy relationship can only be achieved if many good things are happening for you and your partner simultaneously. In a simpler sense, discoveries about your relationship should be made first before you come up with a script that can help achieve this goal.

One common issue that you or your partner might have that can destroy the goal of building a healthy relationship is jealousy. If such is observed in your relationship, this sample script can help both of you.

- Setup phrase: Even if I feel jealous that my partner is with ____ (the name of the person whom you feel jealous of), I completely love and accept myself.
- TH – I understand that all of this…
- EB – …is part of being in a romantic relationship…
- SE – …and this may only be a test…
- UE – …to see if I have trust in my partner.

- UN – I also understand…
- Ch – …that I can never restrain him/her…
- CB – …from meeting new people…
- UA – …and I can guarantee that…
- TH – …this will not stain or ruin our relationship.

Evaluate if the feelings of jealousy were reduced after reciting the sample script. Feel free to add more rounds until the feeling (as well as the impulse to act out because of this emotion) is subdued.

It would be best if you can get your partner to do the same with you as well as consult an expert to guide you on how both of you can address the issue using EFT. This will be a good ground to address other issues as well (if there are any).

Tapping scripts for making money and reaching your dreams

You can only make more money if you know how to make it work for you and earn more than what you invested. However, most people are hesitant to take the financial risk even if they already have a foolproof plan or a "million dollar idea" that will propel their earnings to new and greater heights.

This tapping script can help reduce or eliminate the inhibitions of these people. By doing so, they will be more open to taking calculated risks as well as give them the strength to make a move and turn their visions into reality.

- Setup phrase: Even if this action can cause me to lose money, I completely love and accept myself.
- TH – This fear of losing money…
- EB – …is what's stopping me…
- SE – …from pursuing this idea that I have in mind.
- UE – You can never blame me for having this fear.
- UN – After all, money is hard to come by these days…
- Ch – …and I may be risking the money…
- CB – …that could have been used for my family's needs…

- UA – …for my savings…
- TH - …and for any unfortunate events.

Evaluate what you're feeling about the issue after one round of tapping. Continue with more rounds of tapping until the severity has significantly decreased. In the final round, you can follow this tapping script as an affirmation:

- TH – I believe that this idea…
- EB – …can make it to the top…
- SE – …and I have to make a small sacrifice…
- UE – …to turn this dream into a reality.
- UN – I have to make my family understand…
- Ch – …that this money to be invested…
- CB – …is to be used for a good cause…
- UA – …for the development of our livelihood…
- TH – …and to achieve this vision that I have.

Eliminating phobias and fears

People have different fears, and these could lead to phobias if they remain unresolved. Aside from the common methods that are used to combat them such as desensitization and exposure therapy, the EFT is a new practice that you can use to counter this problem.

One fear that a large number of people experience would be the fear of speaking in public, or what can be called "stage fright." This sample script can provide you with a good start on how you can address this fear and use it as a pattern to eliminate other phobias that you might have.

Control the physiological symptoms

All kinds of phobia are accompanied by physiological symptoms; after all, it is an intense fear of something. These physiological symptoms (such as pounding heart or getting sweaty even if you're in an air-conditioned room) can make you lose control of yourself and hinder you from acting. However, you have to break through this barrier if you are really determined to eliminate the phobia. By doing so, you'll be able to maintain your composure even when you're facing your object of fear.

You can apply this script to control your physiological symptoms. Remember to tap and recite the script before you go up on stage; the longer the preparation time, the better it is for you. Hence, if you knew that you have to recite in front of a huge audience 5 days from now, you have to start with tapping and reciting the script right at that moment so that when the day for presenting is near, you won't forget the things that you're supposed to say or present. Vividly imagine what it is that you will feel when you're already on stage and about to address the crowd. From there, you can start reciting your setup phrase while tapping your karate chop point.

- Setup phrase: Even if <u>my pounding heart</u> (You may replace it with the physiological symptom that you're experiencing when you're in front of a crowd.) makes me lose control and panic, but I acknowledge what it is that I feel and I completely accept myself.

- TH – I've always hated this feeling.

- EB – It makes me feel afraid…

- SE – …and makes me lose control of the situation.

- UE – This pounding heart…

- UN – …makes me feel dizzy…

- Ch – …and blocks out all my thoughts.

- CB – I can't say what I have to say.

- UA – It's like as if this fear…

- TH – …is restricting all my actions.

After tapping and reciting the script, evaluate if your feelings towards the issue have decreased. You may focus on working with the other physiological symptoms for the succeeding rounds. In this manner, you can learn how to relax regardless of the physiological symptom that you will experience on the actual day of your presentation.

How to clear other life changes

This issue is different from what was mentioned previously. If the former focused on how you can be less resistant to changes, this issue will focus on how you can overcome the fear of the unknown. In a simpler sense, this tapping script will help you to overcome the habit of over-thinking about unfortunate things that you may experience because of the change that the future might bring.

- Setup phrase: Even if I don't have the power to directly influence what will happen in the future and make everything happen in my favor, I completely love and accept myself.

- TH – I'm the driver of a large vehicle…

- EB – …stuck in the mud.

- SE – I have the power to steer…

- UE – …but I can't seem to move forward…

- UN – …and make things happen…

- Ch – …just the way I want them to.

- CB – I feel so helpless…

- UA – …that all of my efforts will not…

- TH – …give me any kind of security.

Upon reaching the top of the head, evaluate your feelings towards this issue. You can add scripts as well as do additional rounds along with this sample. For the final round (when your rating for the issue has subsided), you can recite these affirmations.

- TH – This may be the right time…

- EB – …that I allow myself to…

- SE – …get to experience life…

- UE – …without worrying too much…

- UN – …of what could happen in the future.

- Ch – Starting now…

- CB – …I am welcoming whatever change…

- UA – …it is that I'll experience…

- TH – …and embrace it with open arms.

Tapping script to a new you

If you've gotten used to projecting that image for a considerable amount of time, you may find it hard at first to change the way you present yourself. However, you have to consider that for you to be recognized, you have to do it as a whole package – not just on your skills or expertise, but with your looks as well.

This tapping script can help you transform into a new you.

- Setup phrase: Even if the image that I project is not reflective of what I want others to see, I completely love and accept myself.
- TH – Most people never seem to…
- EB – …take me seriously and see me…
- SE – …as an adult and…
- UE – …a competent human being.
- UN – I do not have the same…
- Ch – …sense of style that they do…
- CB – …since I'm not comfortable…
- UA – …projecting an image that is…
- TH – …not natural for me.

Evaluate your feelings regarding this issue after one round of tapping. You can add scripts along with this sample so that you can fully express your situation. Continue with more rounds until your rating is significantly lower. For the final round, you can start with your affirmations.

- TH – I can do something about this.
- EB – I am asking for people's help…
- SE – …on what they think is the right look for me.
- UE – I am experimenting with different styles…
- UN – …to see what will look good on me.
- Ch – I believe that with this effort…

- CB – …I can achieve the right style…

- UA – …that will make me stand out from the rest.

- TH – Be ready for a new me!

There are many more situations where you can apply EFT and implement changes in your life. These scripts will serve as a guide if you or somebody you know would ever want to work on these issues. One good thing about the use of scripts is that they can be tailored the way you want and need them to; after all, it is you who will benefit from the whole process.

Conclusion

This book has presented the importance of tapping as an alternative method to acupuncture in removing the negative energy that is blocking our meridian points. It also highlighted the use of scripts and positive affirmation to ensure that after unblocking our meridian points, positive energy will flow inside our body and implement positive change in our mind and in our life.

Although EFT is not yet recognized as an actual therapy method by medical and psychological practitioners, it would never hurt to try a method that doesn't use drugs and has been hailed by other people as effective in helping them deal with their everyday problems. Because of the benefits that it can give to those who are practicing EFT, it will only be a matter of time before the professionals will deem it as a legitimate form of therapy that will help people in dealing with their problems.

Printed in Great Britain
by Amazon